NAVIGATING VERTIGO WITH CONFIDENCE AND CARE

Empowering Insights And Mastering Life's Twists And Turns For Mind Body Wellness And Good Relaxation

DR. WESLEY IAN

DISCLAIMER

The information in this book is not meant to replace professional medical advice, diagnosis, or treatment; rather, it is meant mainly for general informational reasons. If you have any questions about a medical problem, you should always consult your doctor or another trained health expert. Don't ever discount expert medical advice or put off getting it because of something you've read in this book.

Any negative effects or repercussions arising from the usage of the material provided herein are not the responsibility of the book's author or publisher. It should be noted by readers that the material in this book is not all-inclusive and might not address every facet of the subject. Furthermore, new research may have an impact on how health concerns are understood or treated because medical knowledge is always changing.

No particular test, treatment, method, or product mentioned in this book is endorsed or promoted by the author or publisher. The reader assumes all risk associated with using the information included in this book.

Before making any big decisions regarding your health, it's crucial to speak with a licensed healthcare provider. The relationship between a patient and their healthcare practitioner should not be replaced by this book, nor is it meant to offer medical advice.

The opinions presented in this book are the author's and may not necessarily represent those of the publisher. Any errors, omissions, or inaccuracies in the information in this book are not the responsibility of the author or publisher.

It is recommended that readers independently confirm any information contained in this book and speak with a healthcare provider about their specific medical needs and state of health.

TABLE OF CONTENTS

ABOUT THE BOOK

"Navigating Vertigo with Confidence and Care" is an indispensable tool for those coping with the difficulties caused by vertigo, a disorder that has a major negative influence on quality of life. The book begins with a thorough introduction that explains its goal and highlights how important it is to treat vertigo with caution and confidence. The purpose of this introduction is to get readers ready for the abundance of knowledge and techniques that will come next.

The book begins with an introduction to vertigo, explaining its description, types, typical causes, and triggers. Through a methodical examination of the signs and symptoms of vertigo, it provides readers with a comprehensive grasp of the condition's complex nature and its widespread effects on day-to-day functioning. This basic understanding provides a strong foundation for the in-depth investigation that follows and acts as a springboard for the ensuing chapters.

One of the book's main themes is getting professional aid, which is explained. The value of a medical evaluation, advice on seeing specialists, explanations of diagnostic testing, and the necessity of keeping a personal health record all highlight the book's dedication to enabling people to make knowledgeable decisions about their health.

The book switches gears and discusses coping mechanisms, such as mindful breathing, relaxation methods, physical activities, and nutrition plans designed to reduce vertigo. This section encourages a comprehensive approach to well-being by offering useful methods to manage the difficulties caused by vertigo. Building on this basis, it discusses the psychological aspects of vertigo and provides techniques for boosting self-esteem, controlling worry and fear, setting reasonable objectives, and utilizing available support networks and local resources.

Home safety changes are highlighted, offering readers advice on how to make a vertigo-friendly space, make use of technology and assistive gadgets, and put fall prevention techniques into practice. The book addresses the complexities of dealing with vertigo in particular contexts, like socializing, traveling, and working, and provides customized advice for a range of circumstances.

In managing vertigo,—which is devoted to emotional well-being—highlights the connection between mental and physical health. In addition to addressing emotional difficulties, it also highlights the mind-body connection and looks at counseling and therapy choices. With these realizations, the book promotes a comprehensive approach to well-being while also providing readers with useful tactics. "Navigating Vertigo with Confidence and Care" is a comprehensive companion that offers more than just guidance to individuals who want to take back control of their lives when experiencing vertigo.

CHAPTER ONE

INTRODUCTION TO VERTIGO

COMPREHENDING VERTIGO

The disorienting feeling of spinning or dizziness known as vertigo is a result of a complex and diverse phenomenon involving the interaction of environmental, psychological, and physiological variables. Fundamentally, studying vertigo entails exploring the complex systems that control our equilibrium and spatial orientation.

The brain combines this information to give a smooth impression of our environment, and the inner ear, an essential part of this system, is critical in detecting motion and gravitational forces. As we investigate vertigo, we find that its etiology is not limited to physiological factors; it also involves psychological and situational factors that influence the sensation as a whole.

THE VALUE OF HANDLING VERTIGO WITH CARE AND CONFIDENCE

It is crucial to manage vertigo with assurance and caution since it can have a serious negative influence on a person's everyday activities and general health. Vertigo can impair general quality of life, interfere with daily tasks, and limit mobility. Untreated vertigo has more negative effects than only the physical realm; it frequently leads to increased tension and worry. Thus, learning how to control and lessen the consequences of vertigo becomes essential for those who want to take back control of their lives.

Handling vertigo requires a sophisticated strategy that blends psychological fortitude with medical knowledge. In this situation, confidence results from having a thorough awareness of one's circumstance and from implementing coping mechanisms to deal with obstacles.

People who are skilled in identifying triggers and putting coping mechanisms into place will be more equipped to get through everyday tasks without experiencing the incapacitating symptoms of vertigo. Additionally, self-assurance promotes a proactive outlook, motivating people to consult a doctor when necessary, participate in therapeutic activities, and consider lifestyle changes that improve their long-term health.

On the other hand, care entails having a kind and considerate attitude toward oneself as well as other people who are experiencing vertigo. The knowledge that vertigo may hurt mental health highlights the importance of having a network of friends, family, and medical experts on hand to assist.

Through recognition of the psychological impact of vertigo and the establishment of an atmosphere that encourages candid dialogue, people can develop resilience and surmount the psychological obstacles linked to this ailment.

Deciphering the intricacies of vertigo necessitates a comprehensive comprehension that includes its physiological foundations as well as its wider effects on a person's life. A guiding concept that emphasizes the value of self-awareness, resilience, and a team approach to treating this complex condition is navigating vertigo with confidence and care. In addition to learning more about the complexities of the human vestibular system, our deeper exploration of the subtleties of vertigo reveals the transformational potential of care and confidence in restoring equilibrium and normalcy.

CHAPTER TWO

FUNDAMENTALS OF VERTIGO
VERTIGO DEFINITION AND TYPES

Vertigo is a complicated and unsettling experience that is typified by a delusional sense of motion or spinning, frequently coupled with unsteadiness and dizziness. It is important to differentiate between vertigo and general dizziness since the former is associated with a particular perception of motion, like spinning or tilting, while the latter may include a wider spectrum of unsteadiness. There are several forms of vertigo, and each has unique traits.

Peripheral vertigo is a common type of vertigo that is usually caused by problems in the inner ear. This includes disorders like benign paroxysmal positional vertigo (BPPV), which is typified by fleeting episodes of extreme spinning brought on by particular head motions. Another kind of peripheral vertigo is Meniere's disease, which is characterized by vertigo episodes along with ringing in the ears and hearing loss.

On the other side, issues with the central nervous system, especially the brain, are the cause of central vertigo. This group includes diseases that impair balance and spatial orientation processing centrally, such as vestibular migraines and vestibular neuritis. Determining the precise kind of vertigo is essential for a precise diagnosis and focused therapy.

TYPICAL CAUSES AND INITIATORS

Vertigo can be caused by a variety of things, and knowing these frequent causes and triggers is crucial to managing the condition effectively. Vertigo can result from inner ear conditions such as inflammation or infections that interfere with the vestibular system's regular operation. Head trauma or injury can also harm inner ear structures or interfere with the brain's capacity to interpret signals related to balance.

Vertigo is a side effect of some drugs, particularly those that affect the central nervous system or inner ear. Vertigo symptoms can be made worse by anxiety disorders and stress, underscoring the complex relationship between mental and physical stability.

Furthermore, diseases like hypotension and dehydration can cause dizziness spells, underscoring the significance of general health in preserving equilibrium.

PRECAUTIONARY REMARKS AND INDICATIONS

It's critical to identify the warning signs and symptoms of vertigo to take timely action and enhance quality of life. Vertigo frequently manifests as a spinning sensation, nausea, vomiting, and an overall unsteadiness. People who have disturbed vestibular signals may have involuntary eye movements or nystagmus. Common concomitant symptoms include headaches, light and sound sensitivity, and difficulty concentrating.

Abrupt and severe episodes of vertigo may be warning indicators, particularly if they continue or recur. Severe imbalance, difficulty standing or walking, and loss of consciousness all call for emergency medical care. If there are other symptoms, such as speech problems or hearing loss, it may be a sign of a more serious underlying issue and will need to be thoroughly evaluated by medical professionals.

CONSEQUENCES FOR DAILY LIVING

Vertigo can have a significant negative influence on daily functioning and several facets of an individual's health. People with persistent vertigo may find it difficult to do daily tasks or have a fear of falling, which can limit their freedom and mobility. The resulting stress and anxiety might worsen one's general quality of life by affecting one's ability to engage in social situations, at job, and in leisure activities.

Those who have vertigo find it difficult to drive and operate large machinery, which raises safety problems. Fear of unexpected dizziness attacks might cause social distancing and a loss of interest in previously appreciated activities. Vertigo may be extremely debilitating, and managing its effects often calls for a multidisciplinary strategy that addresses both the physical and emotional elements of the condition with medical intervention, physical therapy, and psychological support.

CHAPTER THREE

OBTAINING PROFESSIONAL HELP

THE SIGNIFICANCE OF MEDICAL ASSESSMENT

It is imperative to seek expert assistance for health issues to ensure one's well-being, and the need for a comprehensive medical evaluation cannot be emphasized. Accurate diagnosis and efficient treatment planning are based on medical evaluations. Obtaining medical attention is crucial for a thorough assessment of an individual's health when they exhibit symptoms like vertigo, fatigue, or spinning.

ASKING A SPECIALIST FOR ADVICE

A vital aspect of the medical examination process is frequently seeing a specialist, especially when treating specialized conditions like vertigo. Professionals with substantial education and background in the identification and management of disorders affecting the neurological system or the ears, respectively, include neurologists and otolaryngologists. Their specific training makes it possible to conduct a more thorough and focused evaluation, which raises the possibility of determining the underlying cause of vertigo.

VERTIGO DIAGNOSTIC TESTS

Diagnostic tests are usually performed as part of the medical examination and are essential in accurately diagnosing vertigo. These examinations are intended to evaluate several health-related factors, including balance, inner ear function, and neurological reactions. Electromyography (ENG), magnetic resonance imaging (MRI), and the Dix-Hallpike maneuver are common diagnostic procedures for vertigo that might provide important information about the possible origins of the condition's symptoms.

ESTABLISHING AN INDIVIDUAL HEALTH RECORD

Making a personal health record is a proactive and self-empowering move for those who are looking for medical assistance. An extensive summary of one's medical history, current prescriptions, allergies, and pertinent lifestyle factors are all included in a personal health record. Throughout the medical evaluation process, healthcare professionals can use this document as a useful tool to help them decide the best course of action based on each patient's distinct health profile.

A medical checkup is quite important, especially if you are experiencing symptoms like vertigo. A specialist visit improves the accuracy of the evaluation, and diagnostic testing is essential for determining the underlying cause of the symptoms. Establishing a personal health record is a proactive step that guarantees a more thorough picture of a person's health status and helps with better communication with healthcare providers. Proactively seeking out expert assistance helps ensure a precise diagnosis and establishes the foundation for a knowledgeable and individualized treatment strategy.

CHAPTER FOUR

COPING MECHANISMS

TECHNIQUES FOR MINDFUL BREATHING AND RELAXATION

Since high levels of stress and anxiety can aggravate symptoms, coping with vertigo frequently entails regulating these emotions. In this sense, mindful breathing and relaxation methods are useful resources. By taking deliberate, deep breaths, one can better control their autonomic nervous system and cultivate a sense of serenity.

Methods like diaphragmatic breathing, which emphasizes taking deep breaths into the abdomen, can be especially beneficial. Stress reduction and relaxation can also be aided by mindfulness meditation, which promotes nonjudgmental awareness of the present moment.

PHYSICAL ACTIVITIES TO REDUCE VERTIGO

Performing particular types of physical activities can help reduce vertigo symptoms. To enhance balance and lessen vertigo, a healthcare provider can prescribe and oversee vestibular rehabilitation exercises that focus on the vestibular system. These exercises, which aim to improve the brain's capacity to integrate sensory information linked to spatial orientation, frequently involve head and eye motions. Furthermore, exercises like yoga and tai chi can enhance general balance and coordination, which helps those who are experiencing vertigo feel more stable.

NUTRITIONAL POINTS TO REMEMBER

Diet is important for controlling vertigo because some meals and drinks might make symptoms worse or less severe. For those who are easily dizzy, eating regular, well-balanced meals helps to keep blood sugar levels steady. Maintaining adequate fluids is crucial since dehydration can make dizziness worse. Since alcohol, caffeine, and sodium can cause dehydration and alter the fluid balance in the inner ear, some people find comfort in cutting back on these substances. Customizing dietary advice to meet specific needs might be facilitated by collaborating with a registered dietitian or other healthcare provider.

VERTIGO AND SLEEP HYGIENE

For those who suffer from vertigo, developing appropriate sleep hygiene practices is essential because sleep disturbances can exacerbate symptoms. Better sleep can be achieved with regular sleep schedules, a cozy sleeping environment, and relaxation exercises before bed. To reduce the risk of positional vertigo, it might be beneficial to elevate the head when you sleep, either with an additional pillow or an adjustable bed. A peaceful nighttime routine and avoiding stimulant like caffeine close to bedtime can encourage sound sleep, which helps with the overall treatment of vertigo symptoms.

A holistic approach to managing vertigo entails implementing a range of coping mechanisms into everyday living. In addition to physical activities designed to target the vestibular system, mindful breathing and relaxation techniques can assist manage stress and enhance balance. Dietary concerns deal with how food and beverages affect symptoms, and excellent sleep hygiene promotes general well-being. People can reduce the negative effects of vertigo on their daily lives and foster a sense of stability and control by incorporating these coping mechanisms.

DEVELOPING SELF-BELIEF AND COMPREHENDING FEAR AND ANXIETY

Gaining confidence starts with having a thorough grasp of fear and anxiety, seeing that they are normal human emotions and frequently act as defense mechanisms. Fear can come in many different ways and be caused by uncertainty, bad experiences, or self-doubt. On the other hand, fear of the unknown and anticipation of future events are common causes of anxiety. Becoming aware of these feelings and their causes is an essential first step toward developing self-assurance. By revealing the layers of fear and anxiety, people can learn more about what causes them and create effective coping mechanisms.

GRADUAL EXPOSURE AND DESENSITIZATION

This technique is essential for boosting self-assurance. By gradually confronting anxieties or difficult circumstances, people can gradually develop resilience. The degree of fear and anxiety decreases when one exposes oneself to the cause of these feelings gradually, which promotes a sense of mastery and control. This approach works especially well at breaking down large problems into smaller, more achievable tasks, giving people the confidence they need to take on bigger issues. Desensitization gives people the ability to step outside of their comfort zones and develop an attitude that values change and flexibility.

SETTING ACHIEVABLE GOALS

People who set attainable goals tend to be more confident. Unrealistic expectations can damage one's self-esteem and cause feelings of inadequacy. People who set reasonable goals for themselves construct a successful road map that supports a healthy self-image. Establishing reasonable goals requires a careful evaluation of one's skills and a dedication to lifelong learning. Recognizing little triumphs along the road gives one a sense of achievement and strengthens the conviction that obstacles can be conquered. Setting goals and going through the process again helps people become more confident because they can see the results

CHAPTER FIVE

SAFETY-RELATED HOME MODIFICATIONS

ESTABLISHING A VERTIGO-FRIENDLY AMBIENCE

Physical space must be carefully considered when designing a home for someone who has vertigo. This can involve selecting flooring materials that lower the chance of slips and falls and offer firm footing, including low-pile carpets or non-slip tiles. Furthermore, reducing clutter and keeping the pathways in the house clear can help create a safer atmosphere for people who are prone to vertigo. Handrails can provide much-needed support and stability when placed strategically along staircases and in other high-traffic locations.

Lighting should also be taken into account because dim lighting might make vertigo symptoms worse. Having enough lighting that is dispersed correctly might make it easier for people to securely navigate their environment. A vertigo-friendly home should have carefully chosen furniture and fittings, minimize abrupt changes in floor level, and use contrasting colors to improve depth perception.

ASSISTIVE TECHNOLOGY AND DEVICES

For those with mobility issues, integrating technology and assistive devices into the home can greatly increase safety and independence. To make daily tasks easier for people with restricted mobility, grab bars, shower chairs, and raised toilet seats can be added in bathrooms. Touch-sensitive faucets and lever-style door handles can help make using sinks and doors easier.

A key component of designing a living area that is accessible is smart home technology. via little to no physical effort, people can regulate lighting, temperature, security, and other aspects of their surroundings via voice-activated assistants and home automation systems. Incorporating sensor-based systems to identify movement and possible threats is part of a proactive strategy to keep a safe home environment.

TECHNIQUES FOR PREVENTING FALLS

Fall prevention is a crucial component of safety changes to a home, especially for those who are more vulnerable to injuries from balance problems or other mobility limitations.

Support is provided by installing handrails along ramps and staircases, and it is crucial to make sure these are strong and securely fastened. Removing trip hazards—like loose carpets or uneven flooring—is essential to reducing the chance of falls.

Arranging furniture and fixtures in a way that makes sense improves mobility and lowers the risk of accidents. Non-slip mats in high-risk areas such as kitchens and toilets help avoid falls even more. Sustaining a safe living environment requires routine house maintenance, which includes looking for loose handrails, uneven flooring, and broken assistive technology.

Designing a house that puts safety first requires a multimodal strategy that takes into account factors including vertigo-friendly architecture, integrating technology and assistive equipment, and implementing efficient fall prevention techniques. By addressing these fundamental ideas, people can benefit from a more accessible and safe living environment that caters to their particular requirements and difficulties.

CHAPTER SIX

HANDLING VERTIGO IN CERTAIN CIRCUMSTANCES

TRAVELING WHEN EXPERIENCING VERTIGO

Handling vertigo while traveling can be difficult and necessitates thoughtful preparation. Selecting modes of transportation that reduce the risk of motion sickness is essential. Choosing smooth-riding transportation options, such as trains or well-kept cars, will lessen the chance of experiencing vertigo attacks.

Choosing a seat above the wings and maintaining eye focus on a single place throughout takeoff and landing can help reduce symptoms when flying. Furthermore, disclosing the illness to traveling companions guarantees a helpful atmosphere, and scheduling regular pauses for relaxation and readjusting can be advantageous.

HANDLING DIZZINESS AT WORK

It takes a calculated technique to manage dizziness while working productively. It's crucial to design an ergonomic office to reduce head motions and eye strain. Stretching exercises and regular breaks help avoid weariness and lower the chance of dizziness. Open communication about the illness with coworkers and managers promotes sympathy and empathy.

Using strategies like the Pomodoro method, which divides work into intervals with brief pauses, can help reduce vertigo symptoms and improve overall work performance in instances where sustained focus is required.

SOCIALIZING AND TAKING PART IN ACTIVITIES

People with vertigo may find it particularly difficult to socialize, but it is still feasible to take part in activities while reducing discomfort. Selecting locations with sturdy flooring and bright lighting helps lessen sensory overload. Vertigo can be controlled by arranging oneself at events so that there are clear sightlines and few visual distractions.

Building a supportive social network involves being transparent with friends and acquaintances about triggers in particular and the need for understanding. A more pleasurable experience can also be achieved by choosing hobbies that allow for breaks and by taking it slow at social events.

HANDLING RECURRING VERTIGO EPISODES

Preparation and coping mechanisms must be used in conjunction to manage abrupt vertigo episodes. Keeping necessary things on hand, including medicine and comfort supplies, guarantees preparedness for unplanned events. Learning mindfulness exercises and techniques like grounded breathing can help reduce the anxiety brought on by vertigo attacks.

It is crucial to have a backup plan in place in case of flare-ups, particularly for finding a calm and secure spot to relax in public areas. Seeking expert assistance to pinpoint triggers and investigate customized coping strategies might enable people to navigate and manage vertigo difficulties with efficacy. Maintaining a healthy and satisfying lifestyle while effectively controlling vertigo flare-ups requires adopting a proactive mindset and building a support network.

CHAPTER SEVEN

MENTAL HEALTH

HANDLING EMOTIONAL DIFFICULTIES

A complicated and multidimensional part of human health, emotional well-being demands thoughtful attention and consideration. Recognizing and comprehending the different aspects that lead to emotional suffering is necessary to address emotional issues. Events in life, interpersonal connections, stress at work, and even innate biological or genetic tendencies may be among these variables. Taking a comprehensive strategy that considers the physiological and psychological dimensions of emotional well-being is crucial.

Developing emotional intelligence is a useful tactic for dealing with emotional difficulties. This entails having the capacity to identify, comprehend, and control one's own emotions in addition to having the capacity to empathize with those of others. Better interpersonal relationships and increased self-awareness can result from developing emotional intelligence. Furthermore, engaging in mindfulness and stress-reduction practices like deep breathing exercises and meditation can be quite helpful in handling emotional difficulties.

OPTIONS FOR THERAPY AND COUNSELING

Therapy and counseling are essential for helping people who are struggling emotionally. These therapy procedures give people a private, secure setting in which to examine and communicate their emotions. Various therapeutic paradigms provide a variety of strategies to address certain emotional disorders. Examples of these include mindfulness-based approaches, psychodynamic therapy, and cognitive-behavioral therapy (CBT).

For example, cognitive behavioral therapy (CBT) aims to promote better cognitive processes by recognizing and altering harmful thought patterns and behaviors. Psychodynamic therapy examines unconscious tendencies and how emotions and behaviors of the present may be influenced by events from the past.

Conversely, mindfulness-based methods place a strong emphasis on developing a non-judgmental awareness of one's thoughts and feelings as well as being present in the moment.

The kind of emotional difficulties being faced, the therapist's experience level, and the client's preferences all play a role in selecting a counseling or therapy program. Building a therapeutic alliance that facilitates the examination and treatment of emotional problems requires that patients and therapists have a good rapport and mutual trust.

THE MIND-BODY LINK IN THE TREATMENT OF VERTIGO

The whole management of vertigo, a disorder marked by a spinning or dizzy sensation, must take the mind-body relationship into account. Even if the inner ear or central nervous system is the source of vertigo, emotional factors have a big impact on when and how severe it is. Vertigo symptoms can be made worse by stress, anxiety, and emotional distress, which can lead to a vicious cycle where the body and mind conflict.

Incorporating mind-body practices can help manage vertigo. Progressive muscle relaxation and guided imagery are two relaxation techniques that can help lower tension and anxiety, which in turn can lessen vertigo symptoms. Furthermore, by helping people reframe unfavorable ideas associated with their illness, cognitive-behavioral techniques might help them adopt a more adaptable and optimistic outlook.

Exercises like tai chi and yoga improve the mind-body connection in addition to improving general well-being. These exercises promote balance and ease stress by emphasizing conscious movement and breath control. Biofeedback, a therapy technique that assists people in becoming aware of and in control of their physiological reactions, particularly those linked to vertigo, may provide relief in some situations.

Fostering holistic emotional well-being involves several related activities, including identifying and resolving emotional difficulties, investigating counseling and treatment choices, and acknowledging the mind-body connection in vertigo management.

www.ingramcontent.com/pod-product-compliance
Lightning Source LLC
Chambersburg PA
CBHW050708250726
48662CB00002B/918